I0428752

Choose To Change:

A Healthy Eating & Dieting Primer

Disclaimer

Every effort has been made to make all aspects, steps, suggestions and tables in this book as complete and accurate as possible. However, no warranty or fitness is implied. The information provided is on an 'as is' basis. The author and the publisher will have neither liability nor responsibility to any person or entity with respect to any loss or damages arising from information contained in this book.

... Dedicated to my brother

for the life battle he lost ...

... Special thanks to Kate for her support, suggestions and discerning eye ...

Quick Start

You are in a hurry. You want to lose some weight right now. If you don't want to spend a lot of time learning how to lose those pounds, if you just want to do it, this chapter provides the steps to get you started right now, today. You can easily start this program by making a few choices and then sticking to your plan.

First you must decide the body weight you would like to attain. That goal determines how much you should eat each day. Whether you use calories, points or some other measurement method, your food intake must be reduced to lose weight.

Once you know how much you can eat and still lose weight, decide how you want to spread food intake across the day, whether you would like to eat three, four, five or six times.

You will monitor your food intake. It is way too easy to forget about the cookie you grabbed or that smoothie you drank if you don't somehow keep track. In 2008, the American Journal of Preventive Medicine published a study showing that participants who kept a log of food eaten, lost twice as much weight as those who did not track food consumed. I've listed references to the study at the end of this book.

The method I offer for tracking food consumption is based on the exchange system originally developed by the American Diabetes Association in conjunction with the U.S. Public Health Service. Though this measurement method was developed for diabetics, it works for anyone. It also helps to minimize consumption of foods that have little nutritional value. Though this system is based on caloric Intake, you can monitor food eaten by counting portions or counting calories. The choice is yours.

The remainder of this chapter walks you through steps to answer the questions posed above. You will thereby be equipped to begin your new healthy eating strategy.

<u>How much do you want to weigh?</u>

Daily caloric intake must align with goal weight, or at least be lower than current consumption. Multiply your goal weight by ten. The result is the number of calories you may eat per day. A goal of 120 pounds equates to 1200 calories each day, 150 pounds to 1500 calories daily, and so forth. Note that I have not included metric equivalents in this book.

While researching the topic of calories, I uncovered other formulae for calculating total daily calories needed to maintain a certain weight. Simplest formulae multiply chosen weight by a number resulting in calories allowed per day, as I've used above. More complex formulae consider age and level of activity in addition to desired weight. When I tried some of these other formulae, I found that each of them resulted in a higher calorie limit for a chosen goal weight. In my experience, a higher calorie limit would result in less weight lost within the same timeframe.

To ease into the process, you might set interim weight goals and decrease food intake gradually over time. Some sources show a caloric intake per desired pound to be higher than ten. To eat more calories, you must exercise enough to burn those extra calories. Ten is a reasonable number for many Americans, given our somewhat sedentary life styles.

How do you want to spend your calories?

A healthy eating plan requires an appropriate mix of carbohydrates, proteins and fats. A 1200 calorie diet should include the following servings: four carbs, five meats, four fruits, five vegetables, two milks, four fats. To be accurate, you need to know how to measure one serving of each food group. Following are rules of thumb as described in the exchange system:

• One carbohydrate serving is one slice of bread, one small dinner roll, half of a burger or hot dog bun, half a cup of peas, corn, beans, or potato. This serving is about 70 calories. Note that starchy vegetables are counted as carbs, not as vegetables. Also, one half cup of ice cream is counted as a carb, Unless it is low fat, the ice cream also contains two fat servings. French fries are counted as one carb serving plus one fat serving for 10-12 of medium size.

• One meat serving is one ounce and about 55 calories. Cheeses are counted as meats. Visually, four ounces of meat is similar in size to a deck of cards. If the meat is high fat, it is counted as two fat servings in addition to the one meat serving per ounce. Cheeses also have fat content that must be assessed and added. Peanut butter is considered a meat due to its protein content.

3

- One fruit serving is a half cup and about 40 calories. A large banana, pear or apple is two servings. A small banana, pear or apple is one serving. These fruits have higher carbohydrate content than others, like peaches or berries.

- One vegetable serving is a half cup and about 25 calories. Since vegetables are lowest in calories, you can eat a lot of them without worry. Remember, though, that this does not include the starchy vegetables that count as a carb serving. Some vegetables are free like celery. Lettuce can be counted as one serving even if you're having more than a half cup; it is that low in calories.

- One milk serving is one cup of milk or yogurt, about 80 calories. If you have skim, no fat need be counted. If you have one percent, count one fat per serving; if you have two percent, count two fats per serving. Whole milk or yogurt is four fats per serving.

- One fat serving can be a teaspoon to a tablespoon depending on the item. Included are salad dressings, butter, nuts, one quarter of an avocado, oils, olives, lard, one slice of bacon, as well as the fat that must be counted for other foods that contain fat. One portion of fat is about 45 calories.

The table below states the carbohydrate, protein and fat content of one serving of each food group as described above.

Food Portion Values

Food	Calories	Carbohydrate grams	Protein grams	Fat grams
Carb	70	15	2	
Fruit	40	10		
Veg	25	5	2	
Meat	55		7	3
Fat	45			5
Milk	80	12	8	

Use nutrition labels on canned, frozen and processed foods for caloric content. Be aware that nutritional value on labels may not be as exact as one might expect.

How often do you want to eat?

You can eat any number of meals each day. Decide what will work for you based on your current eating habits. For example, if you are used to having two meals and two snacks, plan to eat four times a day. Your choice can change as you monitor your efforts. You may decide differently after a week or two. Don't be afraid to change. You will live with these choices for a very long time, for life! Some helpful tables can be found in the next chapter.

What will you eat at each meal or snack?

If you know what type of food you will eat at each sitting, it will be easier to plan ahead. Better planning makes for a higher rate of success. On the 1200 calorie diet eating four times a day, you might have two carbs, one fruit, one meat, one fat and one dairy at breakfast. You could have one fruit, two vegetables and one fat as a snack. Dinner might include one carb, one fruit, three vegetables, four meats and two fats. Last snack would include one carb, one fruit and one dairy. This is but one example of how to spread food portions throughout the day. Try different options over the course of a month to see what works for you. Note that these food portions refer to servings as defined previously.

Monitor your efforts

Tracking food consumption is critical to success. If you don't monitor what you eat, you will happily forget that extra item you had. You will fool yourself into thinking you are meeting your calorie goal ... BUT ... you won't lose weight. You'll be unhappy and decide that no eating plan works for you. SO ... write everything down, each meal, each day. Add up those calories or food portions. This step is most important to your success.

Remember the study. It has been clinically proven that keeping track of food eaten supports higher weight loss. Additionally compelling, if you performed an internet search using the phrase 'diet journal', numerous results would be presented with offerings of diet journals and related instructions. Keeping food diaries has become an accepted, success supporting activity to change to and maintain new eating habits.

If you stay on track, you should see weight loss the first month. It may take a month to see results. An average weight loss of five to ten pounds per month is good. You will plateau at times. Don't lose hope. Just keep to your plan. You will eventually reach your goal weight. Once there, continue your eating plan. You have made a life change. You can and will maintain your healthy weight as long as you do not go back to eating more calories than your body needs.

More things to keep in mind as you walk this road:

- Eat protein at breakfast and throughout the day as it provides long lasting satisfaction. Eat more non starchy vegetables as they are low in calories and also provide satisfaction.

- Get enough sleep. Our bodies need rest to work effectively.

- Allow yourself a treat once in a while. It'll be easier to stick to your plan the rest of the time.

- If you have a bad day, forget about it and get back to your new eating habits the next day. An occasional bad day will not defeat you.

- MOST IMPORTANT, don't give up. Ultimately, giving up is the ONLY thing that CAN and WILL defeat you.

Drill Down

Now you've got the skinny! You know enough to get going. The following paragraphs include additional details to help you. There are tables and facts to use as you define and refine your plan. If you haven't started eating differently because you want to know more, this is where you will learn. The information is organized along the lines of the choices you made in the previous chapter.

The following table includes goal weight, calories allowed and food group portions to healthily consume those calories. The total calories for food portions in each row may not equal the calories number exactly but they are close enough, within 25 calories.

Weight in lbs	Calories	Carbs	Fruit	Veg	Meat	Fat	Milk
120	1200	4=280	4=160	5=125	5=275	4=180	2=160
130	1300	4=280	4=160	5=125	6=330	5=225	2=160
140	1400	5=350	5=200	5=125	6=330	5=225	2=160
150	1500	5=350	5=200	6=150	6=330	5=225	3=240
160	1600	5=350	6=240	6=150	7=385	5=225	3=240
170	1700	6=420	6=240	6=150	7=385	6=270	3=240
180	1800	6=420	7=280	7=175	8=440	6=270	3=240
190	1900	7=490	7=280	7=175	8=440	6=270	3=240
200	2000	7=490	7=280	7=175	8=440	6=270	4=320

As you review the table, note that extra fat in meat, milk or yogurt is not included in these calorie totals. Lean meat and nonfat milk are assumed. When eating medium or high fat meat, 1%, 2% or whole milk,

count the extra fat content of these foods as fat
servings with fat calories.

You can double values in the appropriate row of
the table for a higher goal weight.

When eating canned or other processed foods,
you can determine how to count the food portions using
nutrition information found on the package. The table
on page five, repeated below, shows the breakdown of
calories, carbohydrates, protein and fat for one portion
of each food type. Refer to the food portion definitions
in the previous chapter, pages three and four, as
necessary.

Food Portion Values

Food	Calories	Carbohydrate grams	Protein grams	Fat grams
Carb	70	15	2	
Fruit	40	10		
Veg	25	5	2	
Meat	55		7	3
Fat	45			5
Milk	80	12	8	

How food portions are distributed across the day is
a personal choice. Do what works best for you. Choose
an eating plan you can maintain. Remember that plans
can change. Adjust your plan when the need arises.
The following tables provide examples of how food
portions can be spread across the day for three of the
calorie options in the table on page nine.

1200 Calorie Options

Meals	Carbs 4	Fruit 4	Veg 5	Meat 5	Fat 4	Milk 2
3 meals						
1	1	2		1	1	1
2	2		2	1	1	
3	1	2	3	3	2	1
4 meals						
1	2	1		1	1	1
2		1	2		1	
3	1	1	3	4	2	
4	1	1				1
6 meals						
1	1	1		1		1
2		1	1	1	1	
3	1		1	1	1	
4	1	1	1	1	1	
5		1	1	1	1	
6	1		1			1

1500 Calorie Options

Meals	Carbs 5	Fruit 5	Veg 6	Meat 6	Fat 5	Milk 3
3 meals						
1	2	1	2	2	1	1
2	2	2	2	1	1	1
3	1	2	2	3	3	1
4 meals						
1	2	1	1	1	1	1
2	1	2	1	2	1	
3	1	1	3	3	2	1
4	1	1	1		1	1
6 meals						
1	1		1	1	1	1
2	1	1	1	1	1	
3	1	1	1	1		1
4	1	1	2	2	2	
5	1	1	1	1	1	
6		1				1

1800 Calorie Options

Meals	Carbs 6	Fruit 7	Veg 7	Meat 8	Fat 6	Milk 3
3 meals						
1	2	2	2	2	2	1
2	2	3	2	2	2	1
3	2	2	3	4	2	1
4 meals						
1	2	1		2	1	1
2	1	2	2	3	2	1
3	2	2	3	3	2	
4	1	2	2		1	1
6 meals						
1	1	1		1	1	1
2	1	2	2	1	1	
3	1	1	2	2	2	1
4	1	1	2	3	1	
5	1	1	1	1	1	
6	1	1				1

Remember to add one fat for medium fat meats, and two fats for high fat meats. Add one fat for 1% milk, two fats for 2% milk and four fats for whole milk.

Don't attempt to be super accurate. The goal is to manage food intake, not go crazy counting. Eating fresh or frozen foods is healthier than eating processed foods. Choose low or no salt canned foods. Use fruits canned in juice, not heavy syrup. Fruit juices are concentrated fruits so check the carbohydrate content noted on the nutrition label.

When eating out, make guesses as to the food portions you are consuming. Use your knowledge of the size of one portion for each food group. Make your best assessments, track your intake and enjoy your meal. Again, don't make yourself crazy trying to be completely accurate. You'll develop good judgment over time.

Monitor the food you are eating each day, making a list of consumed portions. If you plan meals by the day and use the previously provided tables to decide menus, you will know that you have met your goal calories without keeping detailed records.

If you want more flexibility, you can list foods consumed each day. Use a log, noting food type and portion eaten. You might use a table like the one at the end of this chapter. Foods consumed for the day are listed with associated nutrition information. Though the foods eaten this day include extra protein, they have lower fat content and the total caloric intake was below goal. As I've said before, don't get mired in details. This day was great, meeting the goals of a healthy eating plan.

Now you've got the tools, food portion definitions and values as well as goal weight caloric needs. Eat yourself to better health with good eating and lower weight. You can find very detailed exchange lists at the Mayo Clinic website, referenced at the end of this book. Other sources are also available. I've included sample blank logs at the end of the book. You may copy them for personal use.

When you are really comfortable with your new eating habits, you can stop logging. BUT, if weight edges up, start logging again. You don't want to erase the strides you have made by losing track of what you are eating!

Sample Daily Food Consumption Log

Goal totals	1200 calories	150 grams carbs	65 grams protein	40 grams fat	4 carb 4 fruit 5 veg 5 meat 4 fat 2 milk portions
1 banana	80	20			2 fruit
1 piece toast, buttered	70 45	15	2	5	1 carb 1 fat
1 egg	55 45		7	3 5	1 meat 1 fat
1 cup fat free yogurt	80	12	8		1 milk
1 cup berries	80	20			2 fruit
salad of 1 ½ cups veg + 1 tbls dressing	75 45	15	6	5	3 veg 1 fat
4 oz low fat meat	220		28	12	4 meat
1 cup veg	50	10	4		2 veg
half cup potato + 1 tbs butter	70 45	15	2	5	1 carb 1 fat
half cup jello	70	15	2		1 carb
1 cup fat free milk	80	12	8		1 milk
1 serving graham crackers	70	15	2		1 carb
TOTALS	1180	149	69	35	

Food Choice Factors

Read the label: Make sure you are getting what you think you are getting. Ingredients are listed in order of content, e.g. first listed is highest percentage of product. For example, is the first ingredient peppers or vinegar on the hot sauce label? Do you want vinegar? Nutrition facts are also listed. Be aware that the rules governing labels are not as exacting as we would like.

Serving Size: Pay close attention to how much you are eating. The obesity epidemic in this country is as much about serving sizes as anything. We are the masters of super sizing all food portions. When reading those labels, make sure you understand the serving size stated. If you are eating more or less than the serving size on the label, adjust the other numbers accordingly.

Fresh or frozen: Minimize your consumption of processed foods. They contain more chemicals and less nutrients, making them less healthy. Choose fresh or frozen ingredients and make your meals. Don't buy prepared foods. You will discover that you can throw a meal together in little time if you've planned ahead.

Whole grain: Determine how the grain is processed from the label. Is whole grain the first ingredient? Has sugar been added? Consider cereals where advertising boasts how healthy they are because they contain whole grains. But grains covered with sugar are not healthy choices. Use cereals without sugar and add fruit to sweeten them.

Organic: The rules for organic foods are not as strict as we'd like. Don't pay the price if you are not sure that the items are truly organic. Again, read labels! Consider the example of a banana. The peel is discarded. Is organic necessary?

Plan: Prepare for the day or week to stay on plan with healthy food choices (really healthy, not advertised healthy). Home preparation with your knowledge of ingredients is best. Eat healthy. Avoid the chemicals in processed foods.

Fat free: Check the label. Has sugar been added to make up for the lack of fat? Our bodies do not need extra sugar. We get enough naturally through fruits and other carbohydrates. Natural fats are much healthier than processed fats of any kind.

Sugar free: Check the label. Has fat been added to make up for the lack of sugar? Our bodies do not need the chemicals of artificial sweeteners or processed fats. Try eating foods without added sugar and enjoy their natural flavors and sweetness.

Natural fats: Use real butter and olive oil. Avoid all those chemically produced and unhealthy margarines and oils. Remember that our bodies need some fat to function effectively.

Salt (sodium): Foods are naturally tasteful. We don't need added salt. If you have the salt shaker at your elbow, try not using it for a week or two. You may never go back to adding salt to everything. Also watch for sodium in other foods. Check the labels.

Sugar versus high fructose corn syrup: It does not matter how refined sugar is presented. Our bodies don't need it. Natural sources of sugar, like fruits and other carbohydrates, provide sufficient sugar. I just read a label for natural peanut butter. Sugar was added; this is not natural or necessary to the product. Be aware and beware!

Sweets and desserts: These foods are nutrition starved. They contain lots of sugar, oil and flour, things we don't need. Minimize your consumption of these items. Have them at mealtime to allow your body to process them more effectively along with the healthy items you've consumed.

Health issues: This eating plan is comprehensive and applicable to anyone. If you have food allergies, you know what to avoid. If you have blood pressure or cholesterol issues, eating healthier and losing weight will positively affect these numbers. If you have diabetes, this eating plan can greatly improve your blood sugar levels. Design your eating plan around any health issues you may have.

Processed foods: Sugar, flour and chemically produced fats are our worst enemies. These items are extremely unhealthy. Yet they are found in most processed foods. Avoid them!

Diet foods: These foods are processed foods. You can prepare your own diet plate using fresh or frozen foods that don't have all those artificial chemicals, oils, sweeteners, non nutritious additions.

Obesity: Recent health reports on TV news shows, in newspapers, in magazines, have the same story. Too many people in the United States are suffering from obesity, diabetes and other health issues that relate directly to eating habits. We've become addicted to fast foods, fast meal preparation, and lots of processed sugars and fats. None of these are good for us. Changing to natural fresh or frozen foods will make a big difference.

Free foods: Foods with no calories: bouillon, broth, chili peppers, cinnamon, club soda, coffee, consomme, cooking spray, extracts (almond, peppermint, vanilla), garlic, herbs, horseradish, hot pepper sauce, lemon juice, pimento, salad greens, spices, tea, tumeric (mustard), vinegar, Worcestershire sauce plus sugar free gelatin, soda, drink mixes, flavored water, tea, tonic water, water, gum.

Non starchy vegetables: These vegetables are low in calories, have no fat, have great nutritional value, and are filling. You can eat lots of them at little cost to your diet plan so they make great snacks. Here is a list, not comprehensive but a great start: amaranth, artichoke, artichoke hearts, asparagus, baby corn, bamboo shoots, bean sprouts, beets, borscht, broccoli, Brussels sprouts, cabbage (bok choy, Chinese, green), carrots, cauliflower, celery, chayote, cucumber, eggplant, green beans, green onions or scallions, greens (collard, kale, mustard, turnip), Italian beans, jicama, kohlrabi, leeks, mixed vegetables (without corn, peas or pasta), mushrooms, okra, onions, pea pods, peppers (all varieties), radishes, rutabaga, sauerkraut, soybean sprouts, spinach, sugar snap peas, summer squash, Swiss chard, tomato (raw, canned, sauce, juice), turnips, vegetable juice cocktail, water chestnuts, wax beans, zucchini.

Feelings Factors

No magic: You must change your eating habits for life. Otherwise you will not keep the weight off even if you lose it. You can never go back to the old ways.

Food for mood: If you are not hungry, try not to eat. Some of us use food as a soother when emotionally off balance. I know I do. If you notice that you are eating when not hungry, find foods that are low in calories, like non starchy vegetables, and eat those when you feel the need to sate a non existent appetite.

Laugh: Laughter is the best medicine. Laugh out loud, at yourself, at jokes, at everything. Laugh often, at work, at play, at meetings, at parties, all the time.

Recreational eating: If you eat to fill time, eat to watch TV, or eat as part of any ritual, look for something else to fill the void. As I've said before, eat because you are hungry, not because you are bored.

My Story

My brother Raoul was diagnosed diabetic at the young age of 27. He was type II in that his body still produced insulin. He was not processing sugar effectively, resulting in less than healthy blood sugar levels. His doctor gave him diet and exercise recommendations to manage his condition without the introduction of medication. Raoul liked his macaroni and cheese, his sweet rolls, his peanut butter and banana or jelly sandwiches, his soda pop. In those days, diet soda pop was hitting the market. He decided he could make the change to drinking diet pop. He did not find ways to change eating habits or to add more exercise to his lifestyle.

As my brother's body was less and less able to cope with the sugar it produced, he was required to start taking pills to manage blood sugar levels. Again his medical advisors reminded him that he should align his eating habits with nutrition recommendations. He was also reminded of the need to include exercise in his daily routine. Raoul's chosen course would only worsen his condition. Sadly, he did not follow a path to check his degradation and control his diabetes without stronger medical intervention. Instead he progressed, like many diabetics, along the path to pills to insulin shots to more insulin in those shots, to more frequent shots, and so it went.

The many issues the body develops when diabetes takes over were happening to my brother. The list is extensive: loss of feeling in extremities, failing eyesight, heart problems, kidney problems, wounds that won't heal or take forever to heal, loss of sexual prowess. This list is not sequenced in any way. It is my brain dump from watching Raoul fall apart little by little. The saddest thing is that once you recognize that your body is deteriorating, that all these things are happening to you, it is pretty much too late. You may slow down or stop the progression but you can't get back what you've lost.

Raoul had a wound on his foot for over a year. Thankfully, his wound doctor kept working with him. He never experienced an amputation thanks to that doctor. He did lose feeling in extremities. He broke his leg and did not know it. He hobbled around for five or six months, falling often, before being diagnosed.

Eventually my brother started dialysis. His kidneys no longer functioned effectively. He also suffered from neuropathy. He might have suffered burns on hands or feet had he not been careful. Think about it! You can't feel hot or cold. You would not know you burned or froze yourself until you saw the resulting mess of your own flesh. Raoul also experienced failing eyesight, heart issues and erectile dysfunction.

In 1990 I was diagnosed as borderline diabetic. By that time, my brother had been experiencing the effects of full blown diabetes for several years. I weighed in at about 225 pounds, carrying that weight around on a 5'3" frame. If it took me five minutes to decide my course of action, it was a lot. All I could think of was my brother's condition, he having just turned 45. I immediately took action.

I am older than my brother, almost 47 at the time I was diagnosed. I am very lucky to have been bestowed with stronger diabetes preventing genes. I also had healthier eating habits, though obviously not sufficient to keep my weight under control or avoid sweets.

My first step was to obtain diet and exercise information from the doctor on the very day of my diagnosis. His nutritionist provided a pamphlet about healthy eating for diabetics. I immediately stopped eating sweets. No more candy. No more sweet rolls, donuts, cake. I was on a mission. I needed to change course and start with what I already knew. The information I received from the nutritionist was the basis upon which I built my detailed plan.

Between June 1990 and November 1991, I successfully dieted to the tune of a 100 pound weight loss. I have shared my success and often been asked how I did it. In those days, I shared my story via notes. Now I'm sharing it through this book.

The information from my doctor was a pamphlet describing a 1200 calorie diabetic diet program based on the exchange lists I described earlier. Use of exchange lists is recommended by the American Diabetes Association and the American Dietetic Association. I developed my personal diet plan from the information in the program. The first and second chapters of this book describe the steps I took.

I maintained a 1000 calorie diet and lost an average of five to ten pounds per month, slow but healthy. I added walking as my exercise. I enjoy walking outside, taking in nature and the sights around me. The walking helped increase my metabolism a wee bit. After reaching my goal, I started eating 1200 to

1300 calories per day. Maintaining the weight I reached (135 146 pounds) required no more than that amount of calories.

This book describes my dieting steps in detail. It's based on my story. Sadly, my brother's story ended in 1998. He paid the ultimate price for his diabetes prone body and lifestyle when he passed away in September of that year at the young age of 53.

Good luck in your endeavors. Do not lose faith if you have a bad day or a bad week. Just go right back to your plan and program. You will reach your goal in the end and be thrilled with your own success.

References

American Diabetes Association, www.diabetes.org

American Journal of Preventive Medicine, Volume 35, Issue 2, Pages 118-126, August 2008. "Weight Loss During the Intensive Intervention Phase of the Weight-Loss Maintenance Trial", Jack F. Hollis, PhD, Christina M. Gullion, PhD, Victor J. Stevens, PhD, Phillip J. Brantley, PhD, Lawrence J. Appel, MD, MPH, Jamy D. Ard, MD, Catherine M. Champagne, PhD, RD, Arlene Dalcin, Thomas P. Erlinger, MD, MPH, Kristine Funk, MS, RD,, Daniel Laferriere, RN, MSN, Pao-Hwa Lin, PhD, Catherine M. Loria, PhD, Carmen Samuel-Hodge, PhD, RD, William M. Vollmer, PhD, Laura P. Svetkey, MD, Weight Loss Maintenance Trial Research Group

Hellmich, Nanci, July 8, 2008. "Using food diaries doubles weight loss, study shows", USA Today. http://www.usatoday.com/news/health/weightloss/2008-07-08-food-diaries%5FN.htm. Retrieved September 6, 2011

Lilly Leadership 1200 Calorie brochure (60-11-0101-2), Eli Lilly and Company, Indianapolis IN, February 1986

Mayo Clinic, www.mayoclinic.com/health

Choose To Change: A Healthy Eating & Dieting Primer

1200 Calorie Daily Food Consumption Log

Goal totals -->	1200 calories	150 grams carbs	65 grams protein	40 grams fat	4 carbs 4 fruit 5 veges 5 meats 4 fats 2 milks
List food eaten	List calorie value of food	List carb value of food	List protein value of food	List fat value of food	List portion value of food
TOTALS					

Choose To Change: A Healthy Eating & Dieting Primer

1500 Calorie Daily Food Consumption Log

Goal totals -->	1500 calories	190 grams carbs	90 grams protein	45 grams fat	5 carbs 5 fruit 6 veges 6 meats 5 fats 3 milks
List food eaten	List calorie value of food	List carb value of food	List protein value of food	List fat value of food	List portion value of food
TOTALS					

Choose To Change: A Healthy Eating & Dieting Primer

1800 Calorie Daily Food Consumption Log

Goal totals -->	1800 calories	205 grams carbs	110 grams protein	55 grams fat	6 carbs 7 fruit 7 veges 8 meats 6 fats 3 milks
List food eaten	List calorie value of food	List carb value of food	List protein value of food	List fat value of food	List portion value of food
TOTALS					

www.ingramcontent.com/pod-product-compliance
Lightning Source LLC
Chambersburg PA
CBHW070246290526
45789CB00004B/1788